The Ultimate No-Point Clean Eating Cookbook 2025

A Nourishing Collection of Delicious Recipes to Fuel Weight Loss, Boost Energy and Support a Cleaner, Healthier Lifestyle

By Author

Dr. Fred S. Rivera

Copyright © **Dr. Fred S. Rivera** 2025

All rights reserved. No part of this publication maybe reproduced, stored or transmitted in any form or by any means, electronic, mechanical, photocopying, recording, scanning, or otherwise without written permission from the author. It is illegal to copy this book, post it to a website, or distribute it by any other means without permission.

Dr. Fred S. Rivera

The moral right to be identified as the author of this work.

TABLE OF CONTENT

TABLE OF CONTENT 3
INTRODUCTION 6
BENEFITS OF NO-POINT CLEAN EATING 7
TIPS & TRICKS FOR NO-POINT SUCCESS 7
ADVANTAGES OF THIS COOKBOOK 8
BREAKFASTS 9
    1. Sunrise Veggie Scramble 9
    2. Zucchini Oatmeal Pancakes 10
    3. Sweet Potato Breakfast Hash 11
    4. Cauliflower "Grits" with Egg Whites 12
    5. No-Point Breakfast Burrito Bowl 13
    6. Apple Cinnamon Baked Oats 14
    7. Avocado & Tomato Breakfast Stack 15
    8. Asparagus & Egg White Muffins 16
    9. Chia Seed Breakfast Pudding 17
    10. Banana-Coconut Breakfast Bowl 18
SMOOTHIES & DRINKS 19
    11. Green Detox Smoothie 19
    12. Tropical Spinach Smoothie 19
    13. Carrot-Orange Zinger Juice 20
    14. Cucumber-Mint Hydration Smoothie 21
    15. Beet & Berry Cleanser 21
    16. Spiced Golden Turmeric Smoothie 22
    17. Blueberry Ginger Gut-Healer 23
    18. Celery & Green Apple Refresher 23
    19. Strawberry-Lime Protein Shake 24
    20. Pineapple-Cucumber Cool Down 25
SOUPS & STEWS 26
    21. Hearty Lentil & Kale Stew 26
    22. Spiced Carrot-Ginger Soup 27
    23. Tomato Basil Detox Soup 28
    24. Mushroom & Barley Clean Soup 29
    25. Zoodle Minestrone 30
    26. Cauliflower & Garlic Soup 31
    27. Spicy Veggie Chili 32
    28. Spinach & White Bean Broth 33
    29. Sweet Potato-Coconut Curry Soup 34
    30. Summer Squash Soup 35
SALADS & BOWLS 36

31. Rainbow Quinoa Veggie Bowl 36
32. Mediterranean Chickpea Salad 36
33. Crunchy Cabbage Detox Slaw 37
34. Avocado & Mango Salsa Salad 38
35. Grilled Zucchini Quinoa Toss 38
36. Kale & Apple Clean Salad 39
37. Spaghetti Squash Taco Bowl 40
38. Asian Cucumber Sesame Salad 41
39. Roasted Veggie Power Bowl 41
40. Citrus Beet & Spinach Salad 42

MAIN DISHES 43

41. Lemon Herb Grilled Chicken 43
42. Balsamic Veggie Stir-Fry 44
43. Zucchini Noodle Primavera 45
44. Garlic Lime Baked Salmon 46
45. Eggplant & Tomato Stack 47
46. Southwest Black Bean Skillet 48
47. Cauliflower Chickpea Curry 49
48. Spaghetti Squash Pad Thai 50
49. Herb-Crusted Tilapia 51
50. Stuffed Bell Peppers with Quinoa 52

SIDE DISHES 53

51. Garlic Roasted Brussels Sprouts 53
52. Cucumber & Dill Salad 54
53. Sautéed Rainbow Chard 54
54. Turmeric Cauliflower Rice 55
55. Grilled Portobello Mushrooms 56
56. Lemon-Garlic Green Beans 56
57. Apple Cider Cabbage Slaw 57
58. Roasted Carrots with Thyme 58
59. Zesty Tomato & Avocado Salsa 58
60. Crunchy Radish Slaw 59

SNACKS & LIGHT BITES 60

61. Bell Pepper Nacho Bites 60
62. Sea Salt Kale Chips 61
63. Stuffed Mini Cucumbers 61
64. Baked Spiced Apple Slices 62
65. Roasted Chickpeas with Cumin 63
66. Crunchy Veggie Sticks & Hummus 64
67. Tomato Basil Zucchini Bites 64
68. Cabbage Wrap Veggie Rolls 65
69. Spicy Roasted Edamame 66
70. Split Pears with Cinnamon 66

SAUCES, DIPS & DRESSINGS 67

- 71. Creamy Avocado Cilantro Sauce 67
- 72. No-Oil Balsamic Vinaigrette 68
- 73. Roasted Red Pepper Hummus 68
- 74. Lemon-Tahini Dressing 69
- 75. Tomato Basil Salsa Fresca 70
- 76. Garlic-Cucumber Yogurt Dip 70
- 77. Mango Jalapeño Chutney 71
- 78. Creamy Dill Veggie Dip 72
- 79. Zesty Chimichurri Sauce 72
- 80. Spicy Green Goddess Dressing 73

CONCLUSION 74

INTRODUCTION

The Ultimate No-Point Clean Eating Cookbook is your go-to resource for fueling your body, changing your habits, and adopting a healthy, energetic lifestyle based on whole foods. This cookbook was made with you in mind, regardless of whether you're new to clean eating or an experienced meal pepper searching for new recipes.

We are all aware of how difficult it may be to strike a balance between the responsibilities of everyday life and a healthy diet. Food becomes more of a chore than a pleasure when you combine it with the stress of tracking, counting, and continuously figuring out what you can and cannot eat. This cookbook can help with that.

The foundation of this book is the straightforward but potent idea that eating healthily shouldn't be difficult, constrictive, or devoid of fun. With the help of these well chosen no-point recipes, you can eat tasty, filling meals that support your health objectives without worrying about the numbers. These recipes blend the clean eating ideas that support your body from the inside out with zero-point meals from well-known weight loss programs (like Weight Watchers®).

The goal of clean eating is to return to the basics: real food that nourishes your body and promotes your optimal health, such as fruits, vegetables, lean meats, legumes, herbs, and spices. It involves substituting colorful, natural elements that complement your body for processed foods, extra sweets, and bad fats. Combining that strategy with no-point tactics gives you the flexibility to eat in excess, feel satisfied, and stick to your diet plan guilt-free.

This cookbook has 80 delectable, filling, and hassle-free recipes that will make eating clean a breeze. Every meal, from nutritious smoothies and invigorating breakfasts to filling soups, tangy salads, flavorful main courses, and gratifying sides and snacks, is:

- Friendly to zero points
- Pure and lightly processed
- Simple to prepare
- Family-friendly and reasonably priced
- Full of taste and nutrients

These dishes are made for everyday appetites, finicky eaters, hectic schedules, and limited funds. You'll always have a dependable, go-to recipe on hand that supports your objectives and keeps you feeling fantastic, whether you're preparing meals for the week, making a quick lunch, or getting together with friends for a nutritious supper.

Along the way, you'll also discover advice on how to create enduring routines, fill your pantry with wholesome necessities, and cultivate a more positive relationship with food that emphasizes nourishment rather than limitation.

This is a transformational tool, not just a cookbook. It's a call to embrace what your body actually needs, simplify your meals, and rediscover the pleasure of eating. These pages are meant to inspire you to cook creatively, eat with confidence, and live each day with purpose and energy.

BENEFITS OF NO-POINT CLEAN EATING

Freedom from Counting & Tracking: No-point meals eliminate the stress of logging everything you eat. You'll enjoy food freedom without compromising on health.

Nutrient-Dense Foods: Each recipe is loaded with vitamins, minerals, fiber, and antioxidants that support energy, digestion, and immunity.

Weight Management Support: These meals naturally promote satiety and portion control, making it easier to lose or maintain weight without feeling hungry.

Sustained Energy & Focus: Clean, whole foods provide steady fuel for your body — no sugar crashes or mid-day energy slumps.

Improved Digestion: Fiber-rich veggies, legumes, and fruits support gut health and keep your digestive system running smoothly.

Reduced Inflammation: Minimizing processed ingredients helps reduce bloating, joint pain, skin issues, and other signs of inflammation.

Craving Control: Whole foods satisfy naturally, helping curb cravings for sugar and processed snacks.

Heart-Healthy Choices: Many recipes are rich in potassium, healthy fats (from avocado, nuts, and seeds), and fiber — all key for cardiovascular health.

TIPS & TRICKS FOR NO-POINT SUCCESS

Meal Prep = Game Changer: Batch cook soups, grain bowls, and sauces on the weekend so your weeknight meals are stress-free.

Flavor with Herbs & Spices: Skip the oil and salt overload — flavor your food with fresh herbs, citrus, vinegar, garlic, turmeric, cumin, and chili.

Hydrate Intentionally: Drink plenty of water and try infusing it with cucumber, lemon, or mint for extra refreshment and detox support.

Stock a Clean Pantry: Keep essentials like canned beans, lentils, quinoa, veggie broth, and no-salt seasonings on hand for quick, healthy meals.

Build a Balanced Plate: Aim for half your plate veggies, a quarter lean protein, and a quarter whole grains or legumes — all zero-point friendly.

Prep Your Veggies: Wash, chop, and store fresh veggies for grab-and-go snacking or quick meal assembly.

Know Your Zero-Point Proteins: Lean poultry, tofu, egg whites, and legumes can be the backbone of a satisfying meal. Rotate them to keep things interesting.

Avoid Hidden Additives: Read labels and avoid ingredients like added sugars, hydrogenated oils, and artificial preservatives — even in "healthy" items.

ADVANTAGES OF THIS COOKBOOK

All Recipes Are Zero Points: No guessing, no calculating. You can eat freely and confidently while staying within your plan.

Every Dish is Clean & Whole-Food Based: Perfect for anyone looking to reset their eating habits, detox gently, or stay aligned with a wellness lifestyle.

Budget-Friendly Ingredients: Made with every day, affordable items — no fancy or hard-to-find foods here.

Quick and Easy Recipes: Most meals take under 30 minutes and require minimal prep or equipment.

Family-Friendly Options: Great for everyone at the table — even picky eaters will enjoy these tasty, wholesome dishes.

Supports Long-Term Wellness: These recipes aren't part of a fad. They're sustainable for life and adaptable to your personal goals.

Versatile & Customizable: Mix and match ingredients, scale recipes up or down, and adjust spices to make every dish your own.

So put on your apron, flip the page, and prepare to be amazed by how tasty clean, pointless eating can be. This is where your happiest, healthiest self begins, and it tastes fantastic.

BREAKFASTS

1. SUNRISE VEGGIE SCRAMBLE

Prep Time: 10 mins

Cook Time: 8 mins

Servings: 2

Ingredients:

- 1 cup of egg whites
- ½ cup of diced bell peppers
- ½ cup of chop-up spinach
- ¼ cup of diced red onion
- ¼ cup of chop-up tomatoes
- ¼ tsp garlic powder
- Salt and pepper to taste
- Cooking spray

Instructions:

1. Before heating a nonstick skillet over medium heat, lightly spray it.
2. Saute the peppers and onions before adding them. Once softened, sauté for three minutes.
3. Once the tomatoes and spinach have been added, continue cooking for an additional two minutes.
4. Garlic powder, salt, and pepper should be added after the egg whites.. Toss to combine.
5. To ensure the eggs are cooked all the way through, toss them occasionally while they cook.
6. Warm it up before serving.

Nutrition Info (Per Serving):

Calories: 90 | Protein: 14g | Carbs: 5g | Fat: 0g | Fiber: 2g

2. ZUCCHINI OATMEAL PANCAKES

Prep Time: 10 mins

Cook Time: 10 mins

Servings: 2 (makes 4 pancakes)

Ingredients:

- ½ cup of rolled oats
- 1 small zucchini, finely grated
- 2 egg whites
- ½ ripe banana, mashed
- ½ tsp cinnamon
- ½ tsp baking powder
- Pinch of salt
- Cooking spray

Instructions:

1. The oats should be ground into flour in a food processor.
2. Mix the oat flour, banana, shredded zucchini, egg whites, cinnamon, baking soda, and salt in a bowl.
3. Bring a nonstick skillet to medium heat and coat it lightly with cooking spray.
4. For every pancake, pour 1/4 cup of batter. Bake for three to four minions on every side.
5. If preferred, serve warm and garnish with fresh berries.

Nutrition Info (Per Serving):

Calories: 120 | Protein: 7g | Carbs: 20g | Fat: 1g | Fiber: 4g

3. SWEET POTATO BREAKFAST HASH

Prep Time: 10 mins

Cook Time: 15 mins

Servings: 2

Ingredients:

- 1 medium sweet potato, diced
- ½ cup of diced bell peppers
- ¼ cup of diced red onion
- 1 garlic clove, minced
- ¼ tsp smoked paprika
- Salt and pepper to taste
- Fresh parsley for garnish
- Cooking spray

Instructions:

1. Grease a skillet that won't stick and set it over medium heat.
2. Stirring occasionally, cook the sweet potato for 5 minutes after adding it.
3. Toss in the peppers, garlic, and onions. Once soft, continue cooking for another seven minutes.
4. Paprika, salt, and pepper can be used for seasoning.
5. Add the parsley as a garnish and serve.

Nutrition Info (Per Serving):

Calories: 110 | Protein: 2g | Carbs: 22g | Fat: 1g | Fiber: 4g

4. CAULIFLOWER "GRITS" WITH EGG WHITES

Prep Time: 10 mins

Cook Time: 10 mins

Servings: 2

Ingredients:

- 2 cups of riced cauliflower
- ½ cup of unsweetened almond milk
- 1 tbsp nutritional yeast (non-compulsory)
- 1 cup of egg whites
- ¼ tsp garlic powder
- Salt and pepper to taste
- Chop-up chives for garnish
- Cooking spray

Instructions:

1. Warm the almond milk and cauliflower rice in a skillet over medium heat. Turn the heat down to low and simmer for five minutes.
2. Garlic powder and nutritional yeast should be mixed in after salt and pepper have been added. Remove from heat and let cool.
3. After spraying a skillet, fry the egg whites until they set.
4. Cauliflower grits are a delicious addition to scrambled egg whites.
5. Serve immediately after garnishing with chives.

Nutrition Info (Per Serving):

Calories: 95 | Protein: 13g | Carbs: 5g | Fat: 1g | Fiber: 2g

5. NO-POINT BREAKFAST BURRITO BOWL

Prep Time: 10 mins

Cook Time: 10 mins

Servings: 2

Ingredients:

- 1 cup of egg whites
- ½ cup of black beans
- ½ cup of diced tomatoes
- ½ cup of diced bell peppers
- ¼ cup of diced red onion
- ½ cup of cauliflower rice
- ¼ tsp cumin
- ¼ tsp chili powder
- Fresh cilantro, chop-up
- Lime wedges (non-compulsory)
- Cooking spray

Instructions:

1. Coat the skillet with spray oil and sauté the cauliflower rice for five minutes with the chili powder and cumin.
2. Until they are hard, fry the egg whites in a separate skillet.
3. Arrange the following ingredients in a bowl: cauliflower rice, green beans, egg whites, tomatoes, onion, and peppers.
4. Add lime wedges and cilantro for garnish, if preferred.

Nutrition Info (Per Serving):

Calories: 130 | Protein: 14g | Carbs: 14g | Fat: 0g | Fiber: 5g

6. APPLE CINNAMON BAKED OATS

Prep Time: 10 mins

Cook Time: 25 mins

Servings: 2

Ingredients:

- ½ cup of rolled oats
- 1 medium apple, lightly diced
- 1 ripe banana, mashed
- ½ tsp cinnamon
- ½ tsp baking powder
- ½ cup of unsweetened almond milk
- ½ tsp vanilla extract
- Pinch of salt
- Cooking spray

Instructions:

1. Set oven temperature to 375°F. Dot two ramekins with a little spray.
2. In a bowl, combine the almond milk, cinnamon, oats, pear, banana, and salt. Flour the mixture and mix thoroughly after adding the baking powder.
3. Place in baking dishes and cook for 25 mins, or until mixture is brown and firm.
4. Warm it up and top it with an additional diced apple if you like.

Nutrition Info (Per Serving):

Calories: 150 | Protein: 4g | Carbs: 30g | Fat: 2g | Fiber: 5g

7. AVOCADO & TOMATO BREAKFAST STACK

Prep Time: 10 mins

Cook Time: 0 mins

Servings: 2

Ingredients:

- 1 ripe avocado, split
- 2 medium tomatoes, split
- ¼ red onion, thinly split
- Fresh basil leaves
- Juice of ½ lemon
- Salt and pepper to taste

Instructions:

1. Divide the avocado, basil, tomato slices, and onion among individual plates.
2. Pour the lemon juice on top.
3. Add salt and pepper as desired.
4. Quickly prepare and serve.

Nutrition Info (Per Serving):

Calories: 130 | Protein: 2g | Carbs: 9g | Fat: 10g | Fiber: 6g

8. ASPARAGUS & EGG WHITE MUFFINS

Prep Time: 10 mins

Cook Time: 20 mins

Servings: 4 (makes 8 muffins)

Ingredients:

- 1½ cups of egg whites
- 1 cup of chop-up asparagus
- half a cup of red bell pepper that has been chopped
- ¼ cup of chop-up green onions
- ¼ tsp garlic powder
- Salt and pepper to taste
- Cooking spray

Instructions:

1. Set oven temperature to 375°F. Apply cooking spray to the muffin pan.
2. Arrange the asparagus, bell pepper, green onions, egg whites, garlic powder, salt, and pepper in a bowl.
3. Always fill muffin pans three quarters of the way to the top with batter.
4. Set and slightly golden after 18 to 20 in the oven.
5. Allow to cool for a moment before you eat.

Nutrition Info (Per Serving – 2 muffins):

Calories: 70 | Protein: 12g | Carbs: 3g | Fat: 0g | Fiber: 1g

9. CHIA SEED BREAKFAST PUDDING

Prep Time: 5 mins

Chill Time: 4 hrs

Servings: 2

Ingredients:

- 3 tbsp chia seeds
- 1 cup of unsweetened almond milk
- ½ tsp vanilla extract
- ½ ripe banana, mashed
- ¼ tsp cinnamon
- Fresh berries for topping (non-compulsory)

Instructions:

1. Almond milk, chia seeds, vanilla, banana (if used), and cinnamon should all be combined in a container.
2. Allow it sit in the fridge for at least four hrs, preferably overnight, after stirring thoroughly.
3. Serve with a final stir and, if preferred, garnish with berries.

Nutrition Info (Per Serving):

Calories: 130 | Protein: 4g | Carbs: 12g | Fat: 7g | Fiber: 8g

10. BANANA-COCONUT BREAKFAST BOWL

Prep Time: 5 mins

Cook Time: 0 mins

Servings: 2

Ingredients:

- 1 ripe banana, split
- 2 tbsp unsweetened shredded coconut
- ¼ cup of unsweetened almond milk
- 1 tbsp chia seeds
- ½ tsp cinnamon
- 1 tbsp ground flaxseed (non-compulsory)

Instructions:

1. Almond milk, chia seeds, vanilla, banana (if used), and cinnamon should all be combined in a container.
2. Allow it sit in the fridge for at least four hrs, preferably overnight, after stirring thoroughly.
3. Serve with a final stir and, if preferred, garnish with berries.

Nutrition Info (Per Serving):

Calories: 145 | Protein: 2g | Carbs: 19g | Fat: 7g | Fiber: 5g

SMOOTHIES & DRINKS

11. GREEN DETOX SMOOTHIE

Prep Time: 5 mins

Cook Time: 0 mins

Servings: 2

Ingredients:

- 1 cup of fresh spinach
- ½ cucumber, peeled and chop up
- 1 green apple, chop-up
- Juice of ½ lemon
- 1 tbsp fresh parsley
- 1 cup of cold water
- Ice cubes (non-compulsory)

Instructions:

1. Put everything in a blender.
2. Add additional water as needed to blend until smooth.
3. Quickly prepare and serve.

Nutrition Info (Per Serving):

Calories: 50 | Protein: 1g | Carbs: 12g | Fat: 0g | Fiber: 3g

12. TROPICAL SPINACH SMOOTHIE

Prep Time: 5 mins

Cook Time: 0 mins

Servings: 2

Ingredients:

- 1 cup of fresh spinach
- ½ cup of frozen pineapple
- ½ cup of frozen mango
- 1 small ripe banana
- 1 cup of unsweetened coconut water

Instructions:

1. Blend all of the ingredients.
2. Whip until the mixture is velvety smooth.
3. Serve by pouring into glasses.

Nutrition Info (Per Serving):

Calories: 90 | Protein: 1g | Carbs: 22g | Fat: 0g | Fiber: 3g

13. CARROT-ORANGE ZINGER JUICE

Prep Time: 5 mins

Cook Time: 0 mins

Servings: 2

Ingredients:

- 2 medium carrots, peeled
- 2 oranges, peeled and sectioned
- ½-inch piece of fresh ginger
- ½ cup of cold water

Instructions:

1. In a high-speed blender, mix all of the ingredients.
2. Make sure to blend until smooth. If necessary, you can strain it through a fine mesh screen.
3. Enjoy chilled.

Nutrition Info (Per Serving):

Calories: 70 | Protein: 1g | Carbs: 17g | Fat: 0g | Fiber: 2g

14. CUCUMBER-MINT HYDRATION SMOOTHIE

Prep Time: 5 mins

Cook Time: 0 mins

Servings: 2

Ingredients:

- 1 cucumber, peeled and chop-up
- ½ cup of fresh mint leaves
- 1 small green apple
- Juice of 1 lime
- 1 cup of water
- Ice cubes

Instructions:

1. Put everything in a blender.
2. Process till creamy.
3. Chill before serving in glasses.

Nutrition Info (Per Serving):

Calories: 45 | Protein: 1g | Carbs: 11g | Fat: 0g | Fiber: 2g

15. BEET & BERRY CLEANSER

Prep Time: 5 mins

Cook Time: 0 mins

Servings: 2

Ingredients:

- ½ cup of cooked
- ½ cup of frozen mixed berries
- 1 small ripe banana
- 1 tbsp lemon juice
- 1 cup of water

Instructions:

1. Blend all of the ingredients.

2. Mix until combined.
3. Chill and serve right away.

Nutrition Info (Per Serving):

Calories: 85 | Protein: 1g | Carbs: 20g | Fat: 0g | Fiber: 4g

16. SPICED GOLDEN TURMERIC SMOOTHIE

Prep Time: 5 mins

Cook Time: 0 mins

Servings: 2

Ingredients:

- 1 frozen banana
- 1 cup of unsweetened almond milk
- ½ tsp ground turmeric
- ¼ tsp ground cinnamon
- 1 tsp fresh finely grated ginger
- 1 tsp chia seeds (non-compulsory)
- Dash of black pepper
- Ice cubes (non-compulsory)

Instructions:

1. Mix everything in a high-speed blender.
2. Whisk until combined.
3. Serve immediately after pouring into glasses.

Nutrition Info (Per Serving):

Calories: 90 | Protein: 1g | Carbs: 19g | Fat: 2g | Fiber: 3g

17. BLUEBERRY GINGER GUT-HEALER

Prep Time: 5 mins

Cook Time: 0 mins

Servings: 2

Ingredients:

- 1 cup of frozen blueberries
- 1 cup of unsweetened coconut water
- ½-inch piece of fresh ginger
- Juice of ½ lemon
- 1 tbsp chia seeds (non-compulsory)

Instructions:

1. Blend all of the ingredients.
2. Mix until combined.
3. The mixture is best enjoyed immediately after filling glasses with it.

Nutrition Info (Per Serving):

Calories: 70 | Protein: 1g | Carbs: 17g | Fat: 1g | Fiber: 4g

18. CELERY & GREEN APPLE REFRESHER

Prep Time: 5 mins

Cook Time: 0 mins

Servings: 2

Ingredients:

- 2 celery stalks, chop-up
- 1 green apple, chop-up
- ½ cucumber, peeled
- Juice of 1 lemon
- 1 cup of cold water
- Ice cubes (non-compulsory)

Instructions:

1. Blend all of the ingredients.

2. For a smoother consistency similar to juice, blend until smooth. If preferred, filter.
3. Enjoy chilled.

Nutrition Info (Per Serving):

Calories: 50 | Protein: 1g | Carbs: 11g | Fat: 0g | Fiber: 2g

19. STRAWBERRY-LIME PROTEIN SHAKE

Prep Time: 5 mins

Cook Time: 0 mins

Servings: 2

Ingredients:

- 1 cup of frozen strawberries
- 1 cup of unsweetened almond milk
- Juice of 1 lime
- ½ tsp vanilla extract
- 1 scoop plant-based protein powder
- Ice cubes

Instructions:

1. Mix everything until it's creamy and smooth.
2. Serve immediately after pouring into glasses.

Nutrition Info (Per Serving, with no-point protein):

Calories: 100 | Protein: 12g | Carbs: 9g | Fat: 2g | Fiber: 3g

20. PINEAPPLE-CUCUMBER COOL DOWN

Prep Time: 5 mins

Cook Time: 0 mins

Servings: 2

Ingredients:

- 1 cup of fresh
- ½ cucumber, peeled and chop up
- Juice of ½ lime
- 6–8 fresh mint leaves
- 1 cup of cold water
- Ice cubes

Instructions:

1. Put everything in a blender.
2. Whip until the mixture is silky and foamy.
3. If you want it cold, serve it with ice.

Nutrition Info (Per Serving):

Calories: 60 | Protein: 1g | Carbs: 15g | Fat: 0g | Fiber: 2g

SOUPS & STEWS

21. HEARTY LENTIL & KALE STEW

Prep Time: 10 mins

Cook Time: 30 mins

Servings: 4

Ingredients:

- 1 cup of dry lentils, rinsed
- 1 small onion, diced
- 2 carrots, chop-up
- 2 celery stalks, chop-up
- 3 cups of chop-up kale
- 3 garlic cloves, minced
- 1 tsp dried thyme
- ½ tsp smoked paprika
- 4 cups of low-sodium vegetable broth
- Salt and pepper to taste
- Juice of ½ lemon (non-compulsory)

Instructions:

1. Chop the onion, garlic, carrots, and celery and sauté them for 5 min in a big saucepan with a splash of water.
2. Legumes, thyme, paprika, and broth should be added. Heat till boiling.
3. A further twenty-five minutes of simmering should be added after the lentils begin to soften.
4. After 5 min of stirring, the kale should have wilted.
5. Chop some fresh lemon juice and add some salt and pepper. Keep warm before serving.

Nutrition Info (Per Serving):

Calories: 180 | Protein: 13g | Carbs: 30g | Fat: 1g | Fiber: 12g

22. SPICED CARROT-GINGER SOUP

Prep Time: 10 mins

Cook Time: 25 mins

Servings: 4

Ingredients:

- 1 lb carrots, peeled and chop-up
- 1 small onion, chop-up
- 1 tbsp fresh ginger, finely grated
- 2 garlic cloves, minced
- ½ tsp cumin
- ¼ tsp ground coriander
- 4 cups of low-sodium vegetable broth
- Salt and pepper to taste
- Fresh parsley for garnish (non-compulsory)

Instructions:

1. Toss the ginger, garlic, and onion with a little water and cook in a large saucepan for 5 mins.
2. Carrots, cumin, cilantro, and broth should be added.
3. Simmer, covered, for 20 mins, or until carrots are tender.
4. Combine all of the ingredients and puree them with an immersion blender.
5. Add salt and pepper to taste, then top with chop-up parsley before serving.

Nutrition Info (Per Serving):

Calories: 90 | Protein: 2g | Carbs: 20g | Fat: 0g | Fiber: 5g

23. TOMATO BASIL DETOX SOUP

Prep Time: 10 mins

Cook Time: 25 mins

Servings: 4

Ingredients:

- 1 small onion, chop-up
- 2 garlic cloves, minced
- 4 cups of chop-up tomatoes
- 2 cups of low-sodium vegetable broth
- 1 cup of chop-up zucchini
- ½ cup of chop-up carrots
- 1 tsp dried basil
- Salt and pepper to taste
- Fresh basil for garnish

Instructions:

1. Gently cook the garlic and onion in a saucepan with a little water until they are tender.
2. The zucchini, carrots, tomatoes, broth, and basil can be added at this point.
3. Simmer, covered, for 20–25 min after bringing to a boil.
4. For a smoother texture, you can blend the soup if you choose.
5. Sprinkle some salt and pepper on top. Sprig some fresh basil on top.

Nutrition Info (Per Serving):

Calories: 70 | Protein: 3g | Carbs: 15g | Fat: 0g | Fiber: 4g

24. MUSHROOM & BARLEY CLEAN SOUP

Prep Time: 10 mins

Cook Time: 35 mins

Servings: 4

Ingredients:

- 1 cup of mushrooms, split
- ½ cup of pearl barley
- 1 small onion, chop-up
- 2 garlic cloves, minced
- 2 carrots, chop-up
- 2 celery stalks, chop-up
- 4 cups of low-sodium vegetable broth
- 1 tsp thyme
- Salt and pepper to taste

Instructions:

1. Saute the garlic, mushrooms, and onion in a saucepan with a splash of water for 5 mins.
2. Pour in the broth and stir in the barley, thyme, carrots, celery, and celery.
3. The barley needs 30–35 min a simmer after being brought to a boil.
4. Serve immediately after seasoning with salt and pepper.

Nutrition Info (Per Serving):

Calories: 160 | Protein: 6g | Carbs: 33g | Fat: 1g | Fiber: 6g

25. ZOODLE MINESTRONE

Prep Time: 10 mins

Cook Time: 20 mins

Servings: 4

Ingredients:

- 1 zucchini, spiralized into noodles
- 1 small onion, diced
- 1 carrot, chop-up
- 1 celery stalk, chop-up
- Half a cup of green beans, finely chopped
- 1 cup of chop-up tomatoes
- 3 cups of low-sodium vegetable broth
- 1 tsp Italian seasoning
- 1 garlic clove, minced
- Salt and pepper to taste
- Fresh parsley (non-compulsory)

Instructions:

1. Chop the onion, garlic, carrot, and celery and sauté them for 5 minutes in a saucepan with a splash of water.
2. Toss in the green beans, tomatoes, broth, and Italian spice blend.
3. Reduce heat and simmer for 15 minor until vegetables are soft.
4. Cook the zucchini noodles for two or three minutes, or until they are just soft.
5. To taste, add salt and pepper and, if preferred, sprinkle with chop-up parsley.

Nutrition Info (Per Serving):

Calories: 60 | Protein: 2g | Carbs: 13g | Fat: 0g | Fiber: 4g

26. CAULIFLOWER & GARLIC SOUP

Prep Time: 10 mins

Cook Time: 25 mins

Servings: 4

Ingredients:

- 1 medium cauliflower, chop-up
- 1 small onion, chop-up
- 4 garlic cloves, minced
- 4 cups of low-sodium vegetable broth
- 1 tsp dried thyme
- Salt and pepper to taste
- 2 tbsp olive oil

Instructions:

1. After the garlic and onion have softened, sauté them in olive oil for 5 min in a big saucepan.
2. After adding the cauliflower, broth, and thyme, stir to combine. Heat till boiling.
3. Simmer, covered, for 20 mins, or until cauliflower reveres tenderness.
4. Smooth out the soup by pureeing it with an immersion blender.
5. Spice it up with salt and pepper before you heat it and serve.

Nutrition Info (Per Serving):

Calories: 90 | Protein: 3g | Carbs: 18g | Fat: 2g | Fiber: 6g

27. SPICY VEGGIE CHILI

Prep Time: 10 mins

Cook Time: 30 mins

Servings: 6

Ingredients:

- 1 medium onion, diced
- 2 garlic cloves, minced
- 1 red bell pepper, chop up
- 1 cup of corn kernels
- One can of diced tomatoes, without salt
- One can of kidney beans should be rinsed and drained.
- One can of black beans should be rinsed and drained.
- 2 tbsp chili powder
- 1 tsp cumin
- 1/2 tsp cayenne pepper
- 3 cups of low-sodium vegetable broth
- Salt and pepper to taste

Instructions:

1. Toss the bell pepper, onion, and garlic with a little water and cook them for 5 in a big saucepan.
2. Toss in the corn, tomatoes, beans, cumin, cayenne, chili powder, and vegetable broth. Mix by stirring.
3. Simmer for 25 min after bringing to a boil.
4. Season with pepper and salt while still hot from the grill.

Nutrition Info (Per Serving):

Calories: 170 | Protein: 9g | Carbs: 30g | Fat: 1g | Fiber: 9g

28. SPINACH & WHITE BEAN BROTH

Prep Time: 10 mins

Cook Time: 15 mins

Servings: 4

Ingredients:

- 4 cups of fresh spinach
- A can of white beans should be rinsed and drained.
- 1 small onion, diced
- 2 garlic cloves, minced
- 4 cups of low-sodium vegetable broth
- 1 tsp dried basil
- Salt and pepper to taste

Instructions:

1. To soften, sauté the garlic and onion in a saucepan with a splash of water for about 5 mins.
2. White beans, broth, and basil should be added. Heat till boiling.
3. Hold the lid on for 10 minutes while cooking over low heat.
4. Cook, stirring occasionally, for 2 more mins, or until spinach wilts.
5. Serve immediately after seasoning with salt and pepper.

Nutrition Info (Per Serving):

Calories: 120 | Protein: 7g | Carbs: 22g | Fat: 1g | Fiber: 7g

29. SWEET POTATO-COCONUT CURRY SOUP

Prep Time: 15 mins

Cook Time: 35 mins

Servings: 4

Ingredients:

- Pulled and diced sweet potatoes, two medium-sized
- 1 small onion, chop-up
- 3 garlic cloves, minced
- 1 tbsp fresh ginger, finely grated
- One mild coconut milk can
- 4 cups of low-sodium vegetable broth
- 1 tbsp curry powder
- ½ tsp ground turmeric
- Salt and pepper to taste
- Fresh cilantro for garnish (non-compulsory)

Instructions:

1. Toss the ginger, garlic, and onion with a little water and cook in a large saucepan for 5 mins.
2. Curry powder, turmeric, sweet potatoes, coconut milk, and broth should all be added. Heat till boiling.
3. After the sweet potatoes have softened, reduce the heat to low and simmer, covered, for around twenty-five to thirty minutes.
4. Make sure the soup is entirely smooth by pureeing it with either a regular blender or an immersion blender.
5. Add some taste with salt and pepper, then finish it off with a sprinkle of cilantro.

Nutrition Info (Per Serving):

Calories: 210 | Protein: 3g | Carbs: 35g | Fat: 7g | Fiber: 6g

30. Summer Squash Soup

Prep Time: 10 mins

Cook Time: 20 mins

Servings: 4

Ingredients:

- 2 medium yellow squash, chop up
- 1 small zucchini, chop-up
- 1 small onion, diced
- 2 garlic cloves, minced
- 3 cups of low-sodium vegetable broth
- 1 tsp dried oregano
- 1 tbsp fresh basil (non-compulsory)
- Salt and pepper to taste

Instructions:

1. To make the garlic and onion soften, sauté them in a saucepan with a splash of water for approximately 5 mins.
2. Saute the oregano, zucchini, squash, and broth together. Heat till boiling.
3. Cook the squash until it reaches a softness level, which should take about 15 minutes on low heat.
4. Make sure the soup is entirely smooth by pureeing it with either a regular blender or an immersion blender.
5. Season with salt and pepper to taste and top with fresh basil if desired.

Nutrition Info (Per Serving):

Calories: 70 | Protein: 3g | Carbs: 14g | Fat: 1g | Fiber: 4g

SALADS & BOWLS

31. RAINBOW QUINOA VEGGIE BOWL

Prep Time: 15 mins

Cook Time: 15 mins

Servings: 4

Ingredients:

- 1 cup of cooked quinoa (cooled)
- One cup of red bell pepper, finely chopped
- 1 cup of shredded purple cabbage
- 1 cup of shredded carrots
- 1 cucumber, diced
- 1 cup of cherry tomatoes, halved
- ¼ cup of chop-up green onion
- 2 tbsp fresh lemon juice
- Salt and pepper to taste

Instructions:

1. Throw the quinoa, veggies, and green onion into a big basin and mix well.
2. Finally, add some salt and pepper and squeeze in some lemon juice.
3. Mix well and set aside to cool before serving, if preferred.

Nutrition Info (Per Serving):

Calories: 160 | Protein: 5g | Carbs: 28g | Fat: 3g | Fiber: 6g

32. MEDITERRANEAN CHICKPEA SALAD

Prep Time: 10 mins

Cook Time: 0 mins

Servings: 4

Ingredients:

- The chickpeas should be rinsed after draining.
- 1 cup of cherry tomatoes, halved
- ½ cucumber, diced
- ¼ red onion, lightly chop up

- ¼ cup of chop-up fresh parsley
- 2 tbsp lemon juice
- 1 tsp dried oregano
- Salt and pepper to taste

Instructions:

1. Put everything in a big basin and mix it.
2. Carefully mix by tossing.
3. Pour in the remaining ingredients and wait 10 minutes for the flavors to blend.

Nutrition Info (Per Serving):

Calories: 140 | Protein: 6g | Carbs: 22g | Fat: 3g | Fiber: 6g

33. CRUNCHY CABBAGE DETOX SLAW

Prep Time: 15 mins

Cook Time: 0 mins

Servings: 4

Ingredients:

- 2 cups of shredded green cabbage
- 1 cup of shredded red cabbage
- 1 carrot, shredded
- ¼ cup of chop-up cilantro
- 2 tbsp apple cider vinegar
- 1 tbsp lime juice
- 1 tsp finely grated fresh ginger
- Salt and pepper to taste

Instructions:

1. Mix the cabbage, carrot, and cilantro in a big basin.
2. Mix the ginger, lime juice, vinegar, salt, and pepper in a small bowl and whisk to combine.
3. Toss the slaw with the dressing.
4. Wait for 10–15 min before cutting and serving.

Nutrition Info (Per Serving):

Calories: 45 | Protein: 1g | Carbs: 10g | Fat: 0g | Fiber: 3g

34. AVOCADO & MANGO SALSA SALAD

Prep Time: 10 mins

Cook Time: 0 mins

Servings: 2

Ingredients:

- 1 ripe avocado, diced
- 1 ripe mango, diced
- ¼ red onion, lightly chop up
- 1 tbsp lime juice
- 1 tbsp chop-up cilantro
- Salt and pepper to taste

Instructions:

1. Mash the avocado, mango, red onion, and cilantro together in a bowl.
2. Add salt and pepper, then squeeze lime juice over top.
3. Quickly prepare and serve.

Nutrition Info (Per Serving):

Calories: 160 | Protein: 2g | Carbs: 20g | Fat: 9g | Fiber: 5g

35. GRILLED ZUCCHINI QUINOA TOSS

Prep Time: 15 mins

Cook Time: 10 mins

Servings: 4

Ingredients:

- 2 medium zucchini, split into rounds
- 1 cup of cooked quinoa
- 1 cup of cherry tomatoes, halved
- ¼ cup of chop-up fresh basil
- 2 tbsp balsamic vinegar
- Salt and pepper to taste

Instructions:

1. To achieve a soft and slightly browned texture, grill the zucchini slices for three to four min per side.
2. After the quinoa is cooked, combine it with the cherry tomatoes and basil in a large bowl.
3. Finish the grilled zucchini by drizzling it with balsamic vinegar.
4. Before serving, lightly toss with salt and pepper.

Nutrition Info (Per Serving):

Calories: 150 | Protein: 5g | Carbs: 25g | Fat: 3g | Fiber: 4g

36. KALE & APPLE CLEAN SALAD

Prep Time: 10 mins

Cook Time: 0 mins

Servings: 4

Ingredients:

- 4 cups of chop-up kale
- 1 large apple, thinly split
- ¼ cup of red onion, thinly split
- 1 tbsp lemon juice
- 1 tbsp apple cider vinegar
- Salt and pepper to taste

Instructions:

1. The kale will become tender after one minute of massaging it with the lemon juice.
2. Pare the apple and add the red onion slices.
3. Finish with a drizzle of apple cider vinegar and a pinch of pepper.
4. Lightly mix and serve immediately.

Nutrition Info (Per Serving):

Calories: 60 | Protein: 2g | Carbs: 14g | Fat: 0g | Fiber: 3g

37. SPAGHETTI SQUASH TACO BOWL

Prep Time: 15 mins

Cook Time: 40 mins

Servings: 2

Ingredients:

- 1 small spaghetti squash
- The beans must be rinsed and drained before use.
- ½ cup of corn kernels
- ½ cup of diced tomato
- ¼ cup of chop-up red onion
- 1 tsp cumin
- ½ tsp chili powder
- Salt and pepper to taste
- Lime wedges and fresh cilantro for garnishing

Instructions:

1. Set oven temperature to 400°F. Scoop out the seeds and cut the spaghetti squash in half.
2. To achieve tenderness, roast with the cut side down for 35 to 40 minutes.
3. Transfer the strands to a bowl by scraping them with a fork.
4. Mix black beans, corn, onion, tomato, cumin, and chili powder in a separate bowl.
5. Once the spaghetti squash is added, add salt and pepper to taste. Sprinkle cilantro and lime on top. Plate and serve.

Nutrition Info (Per Serving):

Calories: 180 | Protein: 7g | Carbs: 35g | Fat: 2g | Fiber: 8g

38. ASIAN CUCUMBER SESAME SALAD

Prep Time: 10 mins

Cook Time: 0 mins

Servings: 4

Ingredients:

- 2 large cucumbers, thinly split
- 1 tbsp rice vinegar
- 1 tsp sesame seeds (non-compulsory)
- 1 tsp coconut aminos
- 1 tsp finely grated ginger
- 1 green onion, thinly split

Instructions:

1. Slice the cucumber and mix it with the green onion in a big basin.
2. Blend the ginger, vinegar, and coconut aminos in a little mortar and pestle.
3. Toss the cucumber in the dressing and set aside.
4. Sprinkle some sesame seeds over the dish.

Nutrition Info (Per Serving):

Calories: 30 | Protein: 1g | Carbs: 6g | Fat: 0g | Fiber: 1g

39. ROASTED VEGGIE POWER BOWL

Prep Time: 15 mins

Cook Time: 30 mins

Servings: 4

Ingredients:

- 1 cup of broccoli florets
- 1 cup of cauliflower florets
- 1 red bell pepper, chop up
- 1 zucchini, chop-up
- 1 cup of cooked quinoa
- 2 tbsp balsamic vinegar

- Salt and pepper to taste

Instructions:

1. Get the oven hot, about 425°F.
2. Mix vegetables with balsamic vinegar, and seasonings, and toss to coat. Distribute it across a baking pan.
3. To achieve a browned and tender texture, roast for 25-30 mins.
4. Arrange on top of cooked quinoa before serving.

Nutrition Info (Per Serving):

Calories: 160 | Protein: 5g | Carbs: 27g | Fat: 3g | Fiber: 6g

40. CITRUS BEET & SPINACH SALAD

Prep Time: 10 mins

Cook Time: 0 min (use pre-cooked beets)

Servings: 4

Ingredients:

- 2 cups of baby spinach
- 1 cup of cooked beets, diced
- 1 orange, segmented
- 2 tbsp red onion, thinly split
- 1 tbsp balsamic vinegar
- Salt and pepper to taste

Instructions:

1. Toss the beets, spinach, orange, and red onion in a large basin.
2. Season with salt and pepper, then drizzle with balsamic vinegar.
3. Lightly mix and serve cold.

Nutrition Info (Per Serving):

Calories: 80 | Protein: 2g | Carbs: 17g | Fat: 0g | Fiber: 4g

MAIN DISHES

41. LEMON HERB GRILLED CHICKEN

Prep Time: 10 mins

Cook Time: 15 mins

Servings: 4

Ingredients:

- 4 boneless, skinless chicken breasts
- Juice of 1 lemon
- 2 garlic cloves, minced
- 1 tsp dried oregano
- 1 tsp dried thyme
- Salt and pepper to taste
- Fresh parsley for garnish

Instructions:

1. You need to combine lime juice, garlic, oregano, thyme, salt, and pepper in a basin.
2. For a minimum of half an hr, marinate the chicken in the mixture.
3. Get a grill by heating it over medium-high heat.
4. To get a chicken internal temperature of 165 degrees Fahrenheit, grill it for 6 to 8 minon ever side.
5. Give it a 5-minute rest and top it with some parsley before serving.

Nutrition Info (Per Serving):

Calories: 150 | Protein: 27g | Carbs: 1g | Fat: 4g | Fiber: 0g

42. BALSAMIC VEGGIE STIR-FRY

Prep Time: 10 mins

Cook Time: 10 mins

Servings: 4

Ingredients:

- 1 cup of broccoli florets
- 1 bell pepper, split
- 1 zucchini, split
- 1 cup of mushrooms, split
- 1 red onion, split
- 2 tbsp balsamic vinegar
- 1 tbsp coconut aminos
- 1 garlic clove, minced
- Cooking spray

Instructions:

1. Place a large nonstick pan over medium-high heat until it is hot.
2. Incorporate all the veggies and garlic, and simmer, stirring occasionally with cooking spray or water, for seven to eight minutes.
3. Mix coconut aminos with balsamic vinegar. Before serving, cook the vegetables for two minutes, or until they are just limp and crunchy.
4. Quickly prepare and serve.

Nutrition Info (Per Serving):

Calories: 70 | Protein: 3g | Carbs: 13g | Fat: 1g | Fiber: 4g

43. ZUCCHINI NOODLE PRIMAVERA

Prep Time: 10 mins

Cook Time: 10 mins

Servings: 4

Ingredients:

- 4 medium zucchini, spiralized
- 1 cup of cherry tomatoes, halved
- 1 bell pepper, split
- ½ cup of red onion, split
- 2 garlic cloves, minced
- 1 tsp Italian seasoning
- 1 tbsp lemon juice
- Salt and pepper to taste

Instructions:

1. In a large skillet, sauté the onion, garlic, and bell pepper for three to four minutes over medium heat.
2. Toss in some zucchini noodles and cherry tomatoes.
3. Season with salt, pepper, lemon juice, and Italian seasoning.
4. Once the noodles are soft but not mushy, cook for another four to five minutes.
5. Warm it up before serving.

Nutrition Info (Per Serving):

Calories: 55 | Protein: 2g | Carbs: 10g | Fat: 1g | Fiber: 3g

44. GARLIC LIME BAKED SALMON

Prep Time: 10 mins

Cook Time: 15 mins

Servings: 4

Ingredients:

- 4 salmon fillets
- Juice and zest of 1 lime
- 2 garlic cloves, minced
- 1 tsp paprika
- Salt and pepper to taste
- Fresh cilantro for garnish (non-compulsory)

Instructions:

1. Set oven temperature to 375°F.
2. In a baking dish lined with parchment paper, lay out the salmon fillets.
3. Mince the garlic and toss it with the lime juice, paprika, salt, and pepper in a small bowl.
4. Transfer the mixture to the fish using a brush and distribute it evenly.
5. The salmon should flake easily when tested with a fork after 12–15 min in the oven.
6. Season with cilantro and place a dish on top.

Nutrition Info (Per Serving):

Calories: 210 | Protein: 23g | Carbs: 1g | Fat: 13g | Fiber: 0g

45. EGGPLANT & TOMATO STACK

Prep Time: 15 mins

Cook Time: 20 mins

Servings: 4

Ingredients:

- 1 large eggplant, split into
- 2 large tomatoes, split
- 1 tsp dried basil
- 1 tsp garlic powder
- Salt and pepper to taste
- Fresh basil for garnish (non-compulsory)
- Olive oil spray (non-compulsory)

Instructions:

1. Set oven temperature to 400°F.
2. Before placing the eggplant slices on a parchment-lined baking sheet, lightly coat them with olive oil, if using.
3. Add garlic powder, dried basil, salt, and pepper to the eggplant.
4. Make sure to turn the pan halfway through the fifteen minutes of baking.
5. Stack two or three layers of split tomatoes and cooked eggplant.
6. Put the stacks back in the oven for another 5 minutes to reheat the tomatoes.
7. Finish the look by scattering chopped fresh basil on top.

Nutrition Info (Per Serving):

Calories: 80 | Protein: 2g | Carbs: 16g | Fat: 1g | Fiber: 5g

46. Southwest Black Bean Skillet

Prep Time: 10 mins

Cook Time: 15 mins

Servings: 4

Ingredients:

- One can of black beans should be rinsed and drained.
- 1 cup of corn kernels
- 1 bell pepper, chop-up
- 1 small red onion, chop-up
- 1 tsp chili powder
- 1 tsp cumin
- 1 garlic clove, minced
- Juice of 1 lime
- Salt and pepper to taste
- Fresh cilantro for garnish

Instructions:

1. A nonstick skillet should be heated over medium heat.
2. Toss in the garlic, bell pepper, and onion. Fry for three to four minutes.
3. Incorporate corn, black beans, cumin, chili powder, salt, and pepper. After 8 to 10 min of stirring, the mixture should be cooked through.
4. Serve with a squeeze of lime juice and a sprinkle of cilantro.

Nutrition Info (Per Serving):

Calories: 170 | Protein: 7g | Carbs: 30g | Fat: 2g | Fiber: 8g

47. Cauliflower Chickpea Curry

Prep Time: 10 mins

Cook Time: 20 mins

Servings: 4

Ingredients:

- 2 cups of cauliflower florets
- The chickpeas should be rinsed after draining.
- 1 cup of diced tomatoes
- 1 small onion, chop-up
- 2 garlic cloves, minced
- 1 tbsp curry powder
- 1 tsp turmeric
- ½ cup of water
- Salt and pepper to taste
- Fresh cilantro for garnish

Instructions:

1. To make the garlic and onion soften, sauté them for approximately three minutes in a large pan.
2. Curry powder, turmeric, chickpeas, tomatoes, and broth should be added to the cauliflower.
3. Reduce heat to low, cover, and simmer for 15 to 20 mins, or until cauliflower reveres desired tenderness.
4. Sprinkle some salt and pepper on top. Reheat the meal before garnishing it with cilantro.

Nutrition Info (Per Serving):

Calories: 180 | Protein: 9g | Carbs: 28g | Fat: 3g | Fiber: 7g

48. SPAGHETTI SQUASH PAD THAI

Prep Time: 15 mins

Cook Time: 40 mins

Servings: 4

Ingredients:

- 1 medium spaghetti squash
- 1 cup of shredded carrots
- 1 red bell pepper, thinly split
- 1 green onion, split
- 2 garlic cloves, minced
- 2 tbsp coconut aminos
- 1 tbsp lime juice
- 1 tsp finely grated ginger
- Red pepper flakes (non-compulsory)
- Lime wedges and fresh cilantro for garnishing

Instructions:

1. Set oven temperature to 400°F. After halving the spaghetti squash, scoop out its seeds and roast it with the cut side down for 35 to 40 mins.
2. Squash, once soft, can be forked into strands.
3. Chop the garlic and sauté the bell pepper and carrots in a large skillet for three to four minutes.
4. Along with the squash, lime juice, ginger, coconut aminos, and red pepper flakes, add the lime.
5. Warm through after a good toss. Finish with a garnish of green onions and cilantro right before serving.

Nutrition Info (Per Serving):

Calories: 110 | Protein: 3g | Carbs: 23g | Fat: 2g | Fiber: 5g

49. HERB-CRUSTED TILAPIA

Prep Time: 10 mins

Cook Time: 12 mins

Servings: 4

Ingredients:

- 4 tilapia fillets
- 1 tsp garlic powder
- 1 tsp dried thyme
- 1 tsp dried oregano
- ½ tsp paprika
- Salt and pepper to taste
- Juice of ½ lemon

Instructions:

1. Set oven temperature to 375°F. Scatter parchment paper onto a baking sheet.
2. In a little bowl, combine the paprika, pepper, salt, oregano, thyme, and garlic powder.
3. Coat the tilapia fillets with the seasoning.
4. After ten or twelve min in the oven, the fillets should flake easily.
5. Top with a squeeze of lemon just before serving.

Nutrition Info (Per Serving):

Calories: 140 | Protein: 26g | Carbs: 1g | Fat: 3g | Fiber: 0g

50. STUFFED BELL PEPPERS WITH QUINOA

Prep Time: 15 mins

Cook Time: 25 mins

Servings: 4

Ingredients:

- 4 grape tomatoes, with the seeds removed and the tops cut off
- 1 cup of cooked quinoa
- 1 cup of chop-up spinach
- 1 cup of diced tomatoes
- 1 can (15 oz) black beans, rinsed and drained
- 1 tsp cumin
- ½ tsp garlic powder
- Salt and pepper to taste

Instructions:

1. Set oven temperature to 375°F.
2. Mix the following ingredients in a bowl: quinoa, spinach, tomatoes, black beans, cumin, garlic powder, salt, and pepper.
3. Put the peppers in a baking tray with their stems facing up after stuffing them with the mixture.
4. Place ½ cup of water in the dish's base and then cover it with foil.
5. After 25 mins, the peppers should be soft enough to handle. Warm it up before serving.

Nutrition Info (Per Serving):

Calories: 190 | Protein: 8g | Carbs: 34g | Fat: 2g | Fiber: 9g

SIDE DISHES

51. GARLIC ROASTED BRUSSELS SPROUTS

Prep Time: 10 mins

Cook Time: 25 mins

Servings: 4

Ingredients:

- 1 lb Brussels sprouts, halved
- 3 garlic cloves, minced
- Salt and black pepper to taste
- Olive oil spray (non-compulsory)
- 1 tbsp lemon juice

Instructions:

1. Set oven temperature to 400°F.
2. After you've seasoned the Brussels sprouts with salt and pepper, stir in the minced garlic.
3. Evenly distribute the mixture onto a baking sheet lined with parchment paper and, if desired, gently coat it with olive oil.
4. To achieve a crisp and golden outside, cook, stirring halfway through, for 20 to 25 minutes.
5. If you want, you can drizzle some lemon juice on top before serving.

Nutrition Info (Per Serving):

Calories: 70 | Protein: 3g | Carbs: 13g | Fat: 1g | Fiber: 5g

52. CUCUMBER & DILL SALAD

Prep Time: 10 mins

Cook Time: —

Servings: 4

Ingredients:

- 2 large cucumbers, thinly split
- ¼ red onion, thinly split
- 2 tbsp fresh dill, chop-up
- 1 tbsp apple cider vinegar
- 1 tbsp lemon juice
- Salt and pepper to taste

Instructions:

1. Cucumber, red onion, and dill should all be mixed in a big basin.
2. The vinegar, lemon juice, salt, and pepper should be whisked together in a small basin.
3. Mix well with the salad after adding.
4. Reserve 15 min before serving to allow to chill in the fridge.

Nutrition Info (Per Serving):

Calories: 20 | Protein: 1g | Carbs: 4g | Fat: 0g | Fiber: 1g

53. SAUTÉED RAINBOW CHARD

Prep Time: 10 mins

Cook Time: 8 mins

Servings: 4

Ingredients:

- One bunch of sliced rainbow chard that has been stemmed
- 2 garlic cloves, minced
- 1 tsp olive oil
- Salt and pepper to taste
- Juice of ½ lemon (non-compulsory)

Instructions:

1. Put the garlic in a skillet and sauté it in olive oil over medium heat.
2. Once fragrant, reduce heat to low and simmer for 30 seconds..
3. While stirring often, simmer the chard leaves for 5 to 6 mins, or until they wilt.
4. Taste and season with salt, pepper, and lemon juice before serving.

Nutrition Info (Per Serving):

Calories: 40 | Protein: 2g | Carbs: 7g | Fat: 1g | Fiber: 3g

54. TURMERIC CAULIFLOWER RICE

Prep Time: 10 mins

Cook Time: 10 mins

Servings: 4

Ingredients:

- 1 medium head cauliflower, riced
- 1 garlic clove, minced
- ½ tsp ground turmeric
- 1 tbsp lemon juice
- Salt and pepper to taste
- 1 tsp olive oil

Instructions:

1. Bring a skillet to a medium heat. After one minute, add the garlic.
2. Toss in the turmeric and cauliflower rice. Mixby stirring.
3. To make cauliflower tender, cook for around seven.
4. Before serving, squeeze in some lemon juice and add salt and pepper.

Nutrition Info (Per Serving):

Calories: 45 | Protein: 2g | Carbs: 8g | Fat: 1g | Fiber: 3g

55. GRILLED PORTOBELLO MUSHROOMS

Prep Time: 10 mins

Cook Time: 10 mins

Servings: 4

Ingredients:

- 4 large Portobello mushroom caps
- 2 tbsp balsamic vinegar
- 1 tbsp low-sodium soy sauce
- 1 garlic clove, minced
- Salt and pepper to taste

Instructions:

1. The balsamic vinegar, soy sauce, garlic, salt, and pepper should be combined in a small bowl.
2. Brush the marinade onto the mushroom caps after ten minutes.
3. Bring the grill to a medium-high temperature.
4. Cook the mushrooms for four to five minutes on every side, or until they are soft and blackened.
5. Warm it up before serving.

Nutrition Info (Per Serving):

Calories: 35 | Protein: 3g | Carbs: 5g | Fat: 1g | Fiber: 2g

56. LEMON-GARLIC GREEN BEANS

Prep Time: 10 mins

Cook Time: 8 mins

Servings: 4

Ingredients:

- 1 lb fresh green beans, trimmed
- 2 garlic cloves, minced
- Juice of 1 lemon
- 1 tsp olive oil

- Salt and pepper to taste

Instructions:

1. Cook the green beans in a steamer for four to five mins, or until they are just crisp-tender. Reserve the drained liquid.
2. Put the garlic and either olive oil or a little water in a skillet and set it over medium heat. Fry for a minute.
3. Stir in the green beans and continue to toss for another couple of minutes.
4. After taking it off the stove, squeeze some lemon juice over it. Sprinkle some salt and pepper on top. Warm it up before serving.

Nutrition Info (Per Serving):

Calories: 45 | Protein: 2g | Carbs: 9g | Fat: 1g | Fiber: 4g

57. APPLE CIDER CABBAGE SLAW

Prep Time: 10 mins

Cook Time: —

Servings: 4

Ingredients:

- 2 cups of green cabbage, shredded
- 1 cup of red cabbage, shredded
- 1 carrot, finely grated
- 1 green apple, julienned
- 2 tbsp apple cider vinegar
- 1 tbsp lemon juice
- Salt and pepper to taste

Instructions:

1. Make sure to thoroughly blend the apple, carrot, green cabbage, and red cabbage in a big bowl.
2. Whisk together the lemon juice, salt, pepper, apple cider vinegar, and lemon in a small bowl.
3. Mix the slaw with the dressing after pouring it over it.
4. Give it a 15-minute chill before you dig in.

Nutrition Info (Per Serving):

Calories: 40 | Protein: 1g | Carbs: 10g | Fat: 0g | Fiber: 3g

58. ROASTED CARROTS WITH THYME

Prep Time: 10 mins

Cook Time: 25 mins

Servings: 4

Ingredients:

- 1 lb carrots, peeled and split
- 1 tsp fresh
- Salt and pepper to taste
- Olive oil spray (non-compulsory)
- 1 tbsp lemon juice (non-compulsory)

Instructions:

1. Set oven temperature to 400°F.
2. Season the carrots with salt and pepper, then combine them with the herbs. If desired, drizzle with a small amount of olive oil.
3. Arrange on a baking sheet and roast, tossing halfway through, for 20-25 mins, or until soft and slightly browned.
4. If desired, add a squeeze of lemon juice just before serving.

Nutrition Info (Per Serving):

Calories: 60 | Protein: 1g | Carbs: 13g | Fat: 0g | Fiber: 4g

59. ZESTY TOMATO & AVOCADO SALSA

Prep Time: 10 mins

Cook Time: —

Servings: 4

Ingredients:

- 1 cup of cherry tomatoes, halved
- 1 ripe avocado, diced
- 2 tbsp red onion, lightly chop-up
- 1 tbsp fresh cilantro, chop-up
- Juice of 1 lime

- Salt and pepper to taste

Instructions:

1. Mix the avocado, cilantro, red onion, and cherry tomatoes in a bowl.
2. The zest of one lime should be added with the salt and pepper. Mix gently by tossing.
3. Garnish with and serve right away.

Nutrition Info (Per Serving):

Calories: 80 | Protein: 1g | Carbs: 7g | Fat: 6g | Fiber: 4g

60. CRUNCHY RADISH SLAW

Prep Time: 10 mins

Cook Time: —

Servings: 4

Ingredients:

- 1 cup of radishes, julienned
- 1 cup of shredded carrots
- ½ cup of shredded red cabbage
- 2 tbsp fresh parsley
- 1 tbsp lemon juice
- 1 tbsp apple cider vinegar
- Salt and pepper to taste

Instructions:

1. The radishes, carrots, cabbage, and herbs should be mixed in a big basin.
2. Vinegar, pepper, salt, lemon juice, and vinegar should all be mixed together in a small basin. Whisk to combine.
3. Mix the slaw and dressing and toss until well combined.
4. A little sitting time will allow the flavors to marry.

Nutrition Info (Per Serving):

Calories: 25 | Protein: 1g | Carbs: 5g | Fat: 0g | Fiber: 2g

SNACKS & LIGHT BITES

61. BELL PEPPER NACHO BITES

Prep Time: 10 mins

Cook Time: 10 mins

Servings: 4

Ingredients:

- 2 large bell peppers cut into bite-sized wedges
- Half a cup of black beans that have been rinsed and extracted of their water
- ¼ cup of diced tomatoes
- 2 tbsp chop-up red onion
- 1 tbsp chop-up fresh cilantro
- ½ tsp cumin
- Juice of ½ lime
- Salt and pepper to taste

Instructions:

1. Set oven temperature to 375°F.
2. On a baking sheet, spread out the bell pepper wedges.
3. The black beans, onion, cilantro, cumin, lime juice, salt, and pepper should all be mixed together in a bowl.
4. Spoon the mixture onto the wedges of pepper.
5. Ten minutes in the oven should be enough to heat it through.
6. Enjoy this crispy snack right away for a guilt-free snack.

Nutrition Info (Per Serving):

Calories: 60 | Protein: 3g | Carbs: 12g | Fat: 0g | Fiber: 4g

62. SEA SALT KALE CHIPS

Prep Time: 10 mins

Cook Time: 15 mins

Servings: 4

Ingredients:

- Roughly slice one bunch of stemmed kale into bite-sized pieces.
- Olive oil spray (non-compulsory)
- Sea salt to taste

Instructions:

1. Set oven temperature to 300°F.
2. Thoroughly rinse and pat dry the kale leaves.
3. Evenly distribute the mixture onto a baking sheet. If you're using olive oil, lightly spray it on.
4. Add a pinch of sea salt.
5. Crispiness is achieved after 12–15 min in the oven, with a turn halfway through.
6. Allow the dish to cool completely before consuming.

Nutrition Info (Per Serving):

Calories: 35 | Protein: 2g | Carbs: 6g | Fat: 0g | Fiber: 2g

63. STUFFED MINI CUCUMBERS

Prep Time: 10 mins

Cook Time: —

Servings: 4

Ingredients:

- 4 mini cucumbers, halved lengthwise and seeds scooped out
- ½ cup of mashed chickpeas
- 1 tbsp lemon juice
- 1 tbsp chop-up parsley
- 1 garlic clove, minced
- Salt and pepper to taste

Instructions:

1. Toss the chickpeas in a small bowl with the lemon juice, garlic, parsley, salt, and pepper. Mash to combine.
2. Spoon chickpea mixture into cucumber halves.
3. If you'd like to, chill it for 10 min before serving.

Nutrition Info (Per Serving):

Calories: 50 | Protein: 2g | Carbs: 9g | Fat: 1g | Fiber: 3g

64. BAKED SPICED APPLE SLICES

Prep Time: 10 mins

Cook Time: 25 mins

Servings: 4

Ingredients:

- 2 apples, cored and thinly split
- ½ tsp cinnamon
- ¼ tsp nutmeg
- ¼ tsp allspice
- Juice of ½ lemon

Instructions:

1. Bake at 350 degrees Fahrenheit until stone cold.
2. Incorporate the lemon juice and spices into the apple slices.
3. Line a baking sheet with parchment paper and spread the mixture evenly.
4. Cook for 20 to 25 minutes, turning once halfway through, or until soft and slightly crunchy.
5. Allow to cool a little before you eat.

Nutrition Info (Per Serving):

Calories: 60 | Protein: 0g | Carbs: 16g | Fat: 0g | Fiber: 3g

65. Roasted Chickpeas with Cumin

Prep Time: 10 mins

Cook Time: 30 mins

Servings: 4

Ingredients:

- 1½ cups of cooked chickpeas
- 1 tsp ground cumin
- ½ tsp smoked paprika
- ¼ tsp garlic powder
- Salt to taste
- Olive oil spray (non-compulsory)

Instructions:

1. Set oven temperature to 400°F.
2. Use paper towels to pat the chickpeas dry.
3. Add cumin, paprika, garlic powder, and a little olive oil, if desired, and toss to combine.
4. After brushing with oil, place on a baking sheet and roast for 25 to 30 minutes, stirring the pan occasionally.
5. For optimal crunchiness, let cool before serving.

Nutrition Info (Per Serving):

Calories: 90 | Protein: 4g | Carbs: 15g | Fat: 2g | Fiber: 5g

66. CRUNCHY VEGGIE STICKS & HUMMUS

Prep Time: 10 mins

Cook Time: —

Servings: 4

Ingredients:

- 1 cup of carrot sticks
- 1 cup of celery sticks
- 1 cup of cucumber sticks
- 1 cup of bell pepper strips
- 1 cup of oil-free hummus

Instructions:

1. Get the veggies clean and cut them into sticks before you do anything else.
2. Set the hummus bowl in the middle of the platter and arrange the vegetables on top.
3. As a fast and crunchy snack, serve right away.

Nutrition Info (Per Serving):

Calories: 80 | Protein: 3g | Carbs: 14g | Fat: 2g | Fiber: 5g

67. TOMATO BASIL ZUCCHINI BITES

Prep Time: 10 mins

Cook Time: 10 mins

Servings: 4

Ingredients:

- 2 medium zucchinis, split into
- 1 cup of cherry tomatoes, halved
- ¼ cup of fresh basil, chop up
- Salt and pepper to taste
- Olive oil spray (non-compulsory)

Instructions:

1. Set oven temperature to 375°F.
2. Arrange the split zucchini on a parchment-lined baking pan.
3. Half a cherry tomato, some basil, salt, and pepper should be sprinkled on top of ever.
4. If desired, drizzle with a small amount of olive oil.
5. The zucchini should be soft and the tomatoes should be slightly cooked after 10 min in the oven.
6. Warm it up before serving.

Nutrition Info (Per Serving):

Calories: 35 | Protein: 1g | Carbs: 6g | Fat: 0g | Fiber: 2g

68. CABBAGE WRAP VEGGIE ROLLS

Prep Time: 15 mins

Cook Time: 3 min

Servings: 4

Ingredients:

- 8 large green cabbage leaves
- 1 cup of shredded carrots
- 1 cup of split cucumber
- ½ red bell pepper, julienned
- 1 cup of shredded purple cabbage
- 2 tbsp rice vinegar
- Non-compulsory: 1 tsp sesame seeds

Instructions:

1. If desired, blanch the cabbage leaves in boiling water for one minute to make them tender. Drain and pat dry.
2. Layer the vegetables on top of every flattened cabbage leaf.
3. Add rice vinegar and drizzle.
4. Create a tight roll, similar to a burrito, and then cut it in half.
5. If you'd like, you can top it up with sesame seeds right before serving.

Nutrition Info (Per Serving):

Calories: 45 | Protein: 2g | Carbs: 10g | Fat: 0g | Fiber: 3g

69. SPICY ROASTED EDAMAME

Prep Time: 5 mins

Cook Time: 25 mins

Servings: 4

Ingredients:

- 1½ cups of shelled edamame
- ½ tsp chili powder
- ¼ tsp cayenne pepper
- ¼ tsp garlic powder
- Salt to taste
- Olive oil spray (non-compulsory)

Instructions:

1. Set oven temperature to 400°F.
2. Mix the edamame, spices, and a little oil, if desired.
3. Distribute uniformly onto a baking pan.
4. Cook, stirring once, for 20 to 25 mins, or until crisp and brown.
5. Allow to cool a little before you eat.

Nutrition Info (Per Serving):

Calories: 90 | Protein: 8g | Carbs: 9g | Fat: 3g | Fiber: 4g

70. SPLIT PEARS WITH CINNAMON

Prep Time: 5 mins

Cook Time: —

Servings: 4

Ingredients:

- 2 ripe pears, split thinly
- 1 tsp ground cinnamon
- 1 tsp lemon juice (non-compulsory)

Instructions:

1. Toss split pears lightly with lemon juice to keep them from browning.

2. Distribute the cinnamon evenly.
3. Enjoy as a refreshing and naturally sweet snack when served fresh.

Nutrition Info (Per Serving):

Calories: 60 | Protein: 0g | Carbs: 16g | Fat: 0g | Fiber: 3g

SAUCES, DIPS & DRESSINGS

71. CREAMY AVOCADO CILANTRO SAUCE

Prep Time: 5 mins

Cook Time: —

Servings: 6 (2 tbsp per serving)

Ingredients:

- 1 ripe avocado
- ½ cup of fresh cilantro leaves
- 2 tbsp lime juice
- 1 garlic clove
- ¼ cup of water
- Salt and pepper to taste

Instructions:

1. Blend all of the ingredients.
2. Adding water while combining allows the mixture to be creamed.
3. Season according to your preference.
4. Refrigerate for up to three days if stored in an airtight container.

Nutrition Info (Per Serving):

Calories: 45 | Protein: 1g | Carbs: 3g | Fat: 4g | Fiber: 2g

72. NO-OIL BALSAMIC VINAIGRETTE

Prep Time: 5 mins

Cook Time: —

Servings: 6 (2 tbsp per serving)

Ingredients:

- ¼ cup of balsamic vinegar
- 2 tbsp Dijon mustard
- 1 tbsp maple syrup
- 1 garlic clove, minced
- 2 tbsp water
- Salt and pepper to taste

Instructions:

1. Mix everything in a small bowl set in a lidded jar.
2. Find the right amount of sugar by tasting.
3. Shake well before every use and refrigerate.

Nutrition Info (Per Serving):

Calories: 15 | Protein: 0g | Carbs: 3g | Fat: 0g | Fiber: 0g

73. ROASTED RED PEPPER HUMMUS

Prep Time: 10 mins

Cook Time: —

Servings: 6 (2 tbsp per serving)

Ingredients:

- 1½ cups of cooked chickpeas
- 1 roasted red bell pepper
- 2 tbsp lemon juice
- 1 garlic clove
- 1 tbsp tahini (non-compulsory)
- 2–4 tbsp water
- Salt and pepper to taste

Instructions:

1. Take a food processor and whirl everything together.
2. To achieve the correct consistency, add water as required.
3. You may keep it in the fridge for up to five days if you seal it.

Nutrition Info (Per Serving):

Calories: 45 | Protein: 2g | Carbs: 7g | Fat: 1g | Fiber: 2g

74. LEMON-TAHINI DRESSING

Prep Time: 5 mins

Cook Time: —

Servings: 6 (2 tbsp per serving)

Ingredients:

- 2 tbsp tahini
- 2 tbsp lemon juice
- 1 tbsp apple cider vinegar
- 1 garlic clove, minced
- 3–4 tbsp water
- Salt and pepper to taste

Instructions:

1. Blend all components by whisking them together.
2. Depending on the consistency you're going for, slowly drizzle in water.
3. Apply right away for a maximum of seven days.

Nutrition Info (Per Serving):

Calories: 50 | Protein: 1g | Carbs: 2g | Fat: 4g | Fiber: 1g

75. TOMATO BASIL SALSA FRESCA

Prep Time: 10 mins

Cook Time: —

Servings: 6 (¼ cup per serving)

Ingredients:

- 2 cups of diced tomatoes
- ¼ cup of red onion, lightly chop up
- 1 garlic clove, minced
- ¼ cup of chop-up fresh basil
- 1 tbsp balsamic vinegar
- Salt and pepper to taste

Instructions:

1. In a bowl, mix all of the ingredients.
2. Give it a good 10 minutes to settle so the flavors can combine.
3. Accompany with vegetable chips and enjoy fresh.

Nutrition Info (Per Serving):

Calories: 20 | Protein: 1g | Carbs: 4g | Fat: 0g | Fiber: 1g

76. GARLIC-CUCUMBER YOGURT DIP

Prep Time: 10 mins

Cook Time: —

Servings: 6 (2 tbsp per serving)

Ingredients:

- Half a cup of plain Greek yogurt that is low in fat
- ½ cup of finely grated cucumber
- 1 garlic clove, minced
- 1 tbsp lemon juice
- 1 tbsp chop-up fresh dill
- Salt and pepper to taste

Instructions:

1. Mix everything in a medium basin.
2. Refrigerate for a minimum of 30 minutes to get the best flavor development.
3. Accompany with vegetable sticks.

Nutrition Info (Per Serving):

Calories: 20 | Protein: 3g | Carbs: 2g | Fat: 0g | Fiber: 0g

77. MANGO JALAPEÑO CHUTNEY

Prep Time: 10 mins

Cook Time: 5 mins

Servings: 6 (2 tbsp per serving)

Ingredients:

- 1 ripe mango, peeled and diced
- 1 small jalapeño, seeded and minced
- 2 tbsp red onion, lightly chop-up
- 1 tbsp lime juice
- 1 tbsp apple cider vinegar
- Pinch of salt

Instructions:

1. Heat a small saucepan over medium heat and whisk together all of the ingredients.
2. Mangoes need around 5 in the pan, stirring once or twice, to start softening.
3. Allow it to cool. Chutney can be served chunky.

Nutrition Info (Per Serving):

Calories: 25 | Protein: 0g | Carbs: 6g | Fat: 0g | Fiber: 1g

78. CREAMY DILL VEGGIE DIP

Prep Time: 5 mins

Cook Time: —

Servings: 6 (2 tbsp per serving)

Ingredients:

- Half a cup of plain Greek yogurt that is low in fat
- 1 tbsp lemon juice
- 1 tbsp dried
- ½ tsp garlic powder
- ½ tsp onion powder
- Salt and black pepper to taste

Instructions:

1. In a bowl, add all the ingredients and stir until smooth.
2. Set aside at least fifteen minutes to allow the flavors to blend in the fridge.
3. As a wrap spread, serve with raw vegetables.

Nutrition Info (Per Serving):

Calories: 20 | Protein: 3g | Carbs: 2g | Fat: 0g | Fiber: 0g

79. ZESTY CHIMICHURRI SAUCE

Prep Time: 10 mins

Cook Time: —

Servings: 6 (2 tbsp per serving)

Ingredients:

- ½ cup of fresh parsley
- ¼ cup of fresh cilantro
- 2 garlic cloves
- 2 tbsp red wine vinegar
- Juice of ½ lemon
- 1–2 tbsp water (to thin)
- ½ tsp crushed red pepper flakes

- Salt and black pepper to taste

Instructions:

1. Mix everything together in a food processor.
2. Mix until combined, retaining some texture.
3. To achieve the correct consistency, adjust the seasoning and water.
4. Serve as a garnish for roasted vegetables.

Nutrition Info (Per Serving):

Calories: 10 | Protein: 0g | Carbs: 1g | Fat: 0g | Fiber: 0g

80. SPICY GREEN GODDESS DRESSING

Prep Time: 10 mins

Cook Time: —

Servings: 6 (2 tbsp per serving)

Ingredients:

- ½ avocado
- One and a half cups of low-fat Greek yogurt
- 1 cup of fresh parsley
- ½ cup of fresh basil
- 1 garlic clove
- 1 tbsp lime juice
- 1 jalapeño, seeded
- Salt and pepper to taste
- Water, as needed for thinning

Instructions:

1. Put everything in a blender.
2. If the mixture is too thick, add more water and combine until smooth.
3. To use as a dip, simply drizzle.

Nutrition Info (Per Serving):

Calories: 35 | Protein: 1g | Carbs: 2g | Fat: 2g | Fiber: 1g

CONCLUSION

As you finish reading The Ultimate No-Point Clean Eating Cookbook, pause to consider the significant change you have just made: putting nourishment, balance, and wellness first without feeling guilty or deprived. This compilation of 80 healthy, tasty, and fulfilling recipes is more than just a set of dishes; it's a way of life based on self-care, sustainability, and simplicity.

You've learned how eating can be both delightful and in line with your health objectives over these pages. Every zero-point dish has been carefully crafted to optimize flavor, nutrition, and diversity while maintaining the ease, affordability, and practicality of your daily meals. This cookbook demonstrates that eating properly doesn't need calorie counting or sacrificing flavor, regardless of whether you're on a Weight Watchers® plan, trying to break bad habits, or just want to feel more invigorated and in charge of your food choices.

Eating healthily doesn't have to be scary. Reestablishing a connection with authentic, healthful foods that nourish your body and sustain your life is more important than being flawless or stressing over every bite. You've learned how to turn common ingredients into energizing meals that your entire family will love with dishes that are full of fresh veggies, lean proteins, fiber-rich legumes, antioxidant-rich fruits, and aromatic herbs and spices.

The freedom to enjoy food without fear, tension, or limitations is another aspect of freedom that this book celebrates. You've given yourself the gift of flexibility, ease, and joy in your kitchen by adopting no-point meals. You now have a vast array of choices that can enhance your weight control and wellness journey while adding color, variety, and satisfaction to your plate.

Allow this cookbook to be your dependable partner as you proceed on your journey toward conscious, clean eating. Use these recipes as a starting point to create your own inventive dinners, try new recipes, and return frequently to your favorite recipes. Change the ingredients to suit your lifestyle, add your own personal touches, and—above all—pay attention to what your body requires.

Recall that modest decisions made consistently result in significant transformations. Feeling your best, having more energy, and establishing a healthy relationship with food are all made possible by each clean mouthful you take. One no-point meal at a time, let this be the start of your path to long-term wellness.

We appreciate you bringing this book into your life and into your kitchen. I hope your meals are healthy, your days are full of energy, and your ambitions are always within your grasp.

Printed in Dunstable, United Kingdom